Keto Slow Cooker

Ketogenic Slow Cooker Recipes That You MUST Prepare Before Any Other

(Using 7 Ingredients or Less)

Introduction

Don't babysit food when on the Ketogenic diet when you can use a crockpot to get the job done!

Getting started with the Ketogenic diet is an exciting venture. Think about it; such foods like wheat and various cereals are no longer going to be part of your everyday meals.

Instead, you replace that with meats and different low carb vegetables. It is just as exciting as it is scary though because you now have to consider relying on new ingredients to prepare your meals.

And owing to the fact that preparing meals can take a lot of time, wouldn't it be better if you could just have an appliance that does all the cooking, without you having to 'babysit' the food until it is cooked?

That is the power of the crockpot!

All you need to do is to prepare the ingredients then put them in the crockpot before pressing a few buttons to set how you want it to cook the food. After that, you can leave the crockpot to do its work; you just come back to a warm, freshly cooked meal that you can enjoy!

The best part is that the crockpot can prepare foods for literally every meal; breakfast, lunches, dinners, snacks and desserts! And in this book, I will show you 50+ recipes that you can start with before any other. It doesn't stop there; you can prepare these foods with as little as 7 ingredients or less!

Ketogenic Slow Cooker Cookbook

Let's get started!

Your Free Gifts

As a way of thanking you for the purchase, I'd like to offer you 2 complimentary gifts:

- **How To Get Through Any Weight Loss Plateau While On The Ketogenic Diet:** The title is self-explanatory; if you are struggling with getting off a weight loss plateau while on the Keto diet, you will find this free gift very eye opening on what has been ailing you. Grab your copy now by clicking/tapping here or simply enter http://bit.ly/2fantonpubketo into your browser.

- **5 Pillar Life Transformation Checklist:** This short book is about life transformation, presented in bit size pieces for easy implementation. I believe that without such a checklist, you are likely to have a hard time implementing anything in this book and any other thing you set out to do religiously and sticking to it for the long haul. It doesn't matter whether your goals relate to weight loss, relationships, personal finance, investing, personal development, improving communication in your family, your overall health, finances, improving your sex life, resolving issues in your relationship, fighting PMS successfully, investing, running a successful business, traveling etc. With a checklist like this one, you can bet that anything you do will seem a lot easier to implement until the end. Therefore, even if you don't continue reading this book, at least read the one thing that will help you in every other aspect of your life. Grab your copy now by clicking/tapping here or simply enter http://bit.ly/2fantonfreebie into your browser. Your life will never be the same again (if you implement what's in this book), I promise.

PS: I'd like your feedback. If you are happy with this book, please leave a review on Amazon.

Table of Contents

Introduction   2

Your Free Gifts   4

Breakfast Recipes   13

Breakfast Frittata   13

Bacon Egg Cheese Casserole   15

Breakfast Casserole   17

Easy Breakfast Eggs, Chorizo and Squash   19

Sausage & Egg Breakfast Casserole   21

Easy Crockpot Brats   23

Egg White Vegetable Frittata   25

Yogurt, Kid   27

Santa Fe Omelet   29

Crust-less Broccoli Cheese Quiche   31

Cream Spinach and Mozzarella Quiche   33

Spinach Quiche   34

Sausage Bake   36

Bacon & Egg Casserole   38

Biscuit Breakfast Casserole   40

Frittata with Artichoke Hearts, Red Pepper, and Feta   42

Pizza Casserole   44

Lunch Recipes   46
Shredded Chicken   46
Salsa Chicken   47
Italian Beef   49
5-Ingredient Garlic Balsamic Chicken   51
Steak Fajitas   53
Southern Roast   54
Simple Poached Salmon   55
Taco Chicken   57
Garlic Beef Roast   59
Cheddar Cream of Mushroom Chicken   60
Hawaiian Pulled Pork   62
Buffalo Chicken   63
Caesar Pork Chops   64
Lemon Chicken   65
Balsamic Glazed Short Ribs   66
Chicken Tacos   68

Dinner Recipes   70
Crock-Pot Mississippi Roast   70
Beef Chuck Pot Roast   72
Swiss Steak   74
Garlic Chicken Drumsticks   76
Easy Chili Verde   78

Java Roast Beef	*79*
Kalua Pig	*81*
3 Ingredient Pork Dinner	*83*
Rump Roast with Onions	*85*
Easy Turkey Breast	*87*
Chicken Stroganoff	*88*
Montreal Chuck Roast	*89*
Homemade Italian Beef	*90*
Crust-less Pizza	*92*
Chicken Enchilada Dip	*94*
Whole Chicken	*96*
Chicken Taco Soup	*97*

Snacks and Desserts — 99

Easy Seasoned Pecans	*99*
Peach Cobbler	*100*
Ranch Mushrooms	*102*
Sweet Kielbasa	*103*
Irish Cream Coffee	*104*
Crockpot Brussels Sprouts	*106*
Brownie Pudding	*107*
Steak Bites	*109*
Dulce de Leche	*111*
Crock Pot Candy	*113*

Crème Brûlée *115*

Chocolate Chip Brownie Cake *117*

Cherry Dump Cake *119*

Caramel Apple Spice Cake *120*

Caramel Cake *122*

Buttery Ranch Mushrooms *124*

Conclusion — 126

Do You Like My Book & Approach To Publishing? — 127

1: First, I'd Love It If You Leave a Review of This Book on Amazon. — *127*

2: Check Out My Other Keto Diet Books — *127*

3: Let's Get In Touch — *129*

4: Grab Some Freebies On Your Way Out; Giving Is Receiving, Right? — *129*

5: Suggest Topics That You'd Love Me To Cover To Increase Your Knowledge Bank. — *130*

PSS: Let Me Also Help You Save Some Money! — 131

Copyright 2019 by Fantonpublishers.com - All rights reserved.

PS:

I have special interest in the Ketogenic diet. My wife has been following the Ketogenic diet and I can honestly say that the journey has been amazing. The diet works. And this is why I have committed to writing and publishing as many of the Ketogenic diet books as possible to give readers different options as far as the Ketogenic diet is concerned.

For instance, I have Ketogenic diet books exclusively dedicated for:

- Breakfast
- Main Meals
- Snacks
- Desserts
- Appetizers
- Soups
- Vegetarians
- Crockpot/slow cooker users
- Instant pot users
- Air fryer users
- People who are on the Paleo diet
- People who are following intermittent fasting

- People who are following carb cycling

And much more.

You can check out my [Ketogenic Diet Books fan page shop](#) for more of the books, as I continue publishing more and more. If you want me to add your category of the Ketogenic diet books that I have published so far, make sure to send me a message. I will do the heavy lifting for you and get back to you with a book that you will love.

You could also subscribe to my newsletter to receive updates whenever I have something new: http://bit.ly/2Cketodietfanton.

Breakfast Recipes

Breakfast Frittata

Prep Time: 15 minutes

Cook Time: 2 hours

Total Time: 2 hours 15 minutes

Serves 6

Ingredients

1 1/3 cups cooked sausage

1 teaspoon sea salt

½ teaspoon black pepper

8 eggs

¼ cup diced onion

1 ½ cups of diced red bell pepper

¾ cup of drained frozen spinach

Directions

1. Mix spinach, sea salt, black pepper, eggs, red onions, sausage and red pepper in an oil-greased Crockpot.

2. Cover and cook for 2-3 hours on low or until set.

3. In case you would like to freeze the frittata, cool it for a moment then cut into equal-sized portion.

4. Keep it frozen until ready to serve.

Nutritional Information Per Serving: *Calories 238, Carbs 3g, Protein 20g, Fat 16g*

Bacon Egg Cheese Casserole

Prep Time: 15 minutes

Cook Time: 1 hour

Total Time: 1 hour 15 minutes

Servings: 8

Ingredients

3 green onions, chopped

10 pieces of cooked bacon, chopped

8 ounces of shredded cheddar cheese

1 cup of heavy whipping cream

10 eggs, beaten

1 tablespoon of butter or bacon grease

Salt & pepper to taste

Directions

1. First fry the meat in a skillet until browned then drain it and chop.

2. In a large bowl, crack all the eggs and whisk them together until well beaten.

3. Add in heavy cream along with the cheese. Season the mixture with pepper and salt then whisk to incorporate.

4. Set the crockpot to high setting and then add in bacon drippings or butter. Heat until fully melted.

5. Pour the egg mixture into the Crockpot and sprinkle the crumbled bacon.

6. Cook the casserole on high setting for approximately 1 to 2 hours. You can garnish with chopped onions.

Nutritional Information Per Serving: *Calories 341, Cabs 5.8g, Protein 18.4g, Fat 23.2g*

Breakfast Casserole

Prep Time: 15 minutes

Cook Time: 2 hours

Total Time: 2 hour 15 minutes

Serves: 8

Ingredients

1 (8 ounce) package of Sargento Sharp Cheddar Fine Cut cheese

6 eggs

1 leek, cleaned and cut into half-moon slices

12 fully cooked sausage links, cut into rounds

5 ounces cremini mushrooms, finely diced

1/4 teaspoon salt

10 ounces cauliflower florets

Directions

1. Coat the bottom of a crockpot with cooking spray. In a heat safe bowl, add in the shredded cauliflower and salt.

2. Add water to the bowl to fully cover the bite-sized cauliflower. Put the microwave-safe bowl in the microwave for around 8 minutes or so.

3. Meanwhile, start preparing the leeks, sausage and the mushrooms. Drain the water from barely cooked cauliflower, and add it to the bottom of a crockpot.

4. Distribute the sausage pieces and mushrooms evenly over the cauliflower.

5. Then in a separate bowl, whisk together all eggs and some salt and slowly stir in cleaned leeks.

6. Stir in half of the cheese and reserve the rest. Pour the egg and leek mixture over the cauliflower mixture in the crockpot.

7. Cook the ingredients on high for about 2 to 3 hours. Once the eggs are puffed up, stop the cooking and then sprinkle the rest of the cheese on top.

8. Allow to melt for a couple of minutes then slice the casserole and enjoy. You can season with some pepper if you like.

Nutritional Information Per Serving: *Calories 410, Carbs 7.5g, Protein 26.6g, Fat 35.4g*

Easy Breakfast Eggs, Chorizo and Squash

Prep Time: 10 Minutes

Cook Time: 3-4 hours on high or 6-8 hours on low

Total Time: 3 hours 10 minutes on high to 8 hours 10 minutes on low

Serves 8

Ingredients:

Coconut oil to grease the crockpot and cook onions

1 small to medium butternut squash

1 cup organic lite coconut milk

12-16 eggs

2-4 cloves minced garlic

1 onion diced

1 lb. chorizo sausage

Optional: baby spinach, red pepper flakes

Directions

1. First peel, remove the seeds and chop the butternut squash.

2. Then in a medium skillet, heat coconut oil and add in garlic and onions along with red pepper flakes if you want it.

3. As soon as the mixture begins to soften, add in chorizo. Mix in the spinach and then whisk together coconut milk and eggs.

4. At this point, grease the slow cooker using coconut oil to stop the eggs from sticking.

5. Then put the chopped squash first at the bottom of the crockpot, and follow with the onion and chorizo mix.

6. Flatten the mixture and now pour in the coconut milk and egg mixture.

7. Cook on low setting for approximately 6 to 8 hours or on high for about 3 to 4 hours.

Nutritional Information Per Serving: *Calories 565, Carbs 7.5g, Protein 24.9g, Fat 48.6g*

Sausage & Egg Breakfast Casserole

Prep Time: 10 minutes

Cook Time: 3 hours

Total Time: 3 hours, 10 minutes

Servings: 6 to 8

Ingredients

1/4 teaspoon pepper

1/2 teaspoon salt

2 cloves garlic, minced

3/4 cup whipping cream

10 eggs

1 cup shredded Cheddar divided

1 12- ounce package sausage cooked and sliced

1 medium head broccoli chopped

Directions

1. Coat the interior of your crockpot with grease and then layer half of the broccoli along with half of the cooked sausage and the shredded cheddar cheese.

2. Repeat with the rest of broccoli, cheddar cheese and sausage in the same order.

3. Whisk together whipping cream, eggs, garlic, pepper and salt in a large bowl until well incorporated.

4. Pour the mixture over the layered broccoli and sausage mixture.

5. Cover the ingredients and cook for 4 to 5 hours on low setting or for approximately 2 to 3 hours on high setting.

6. Serve the breakfast casserole as soon as it's set in the center and browned on the edges.

Nutritional Information Per Serving: *Calories 484, Carbs 5.4g, Protein 26.1g, Fat 38.9g*

Easy Crockpot Brats

Prep Time: 15 minutes

Cook Time: 4 hours

Total Time: 4 hours, 15 minutes

Serves 4

Ingredients

2 cups of pepper strips

Dried thyme, basil OR ¼ cup fresh parsley

2 cups of homemade broth

2 medium onions, halved and sliced

2 packages Bison Brats

Coarse sea salt

Favorite hot sauce

Optional

1 cup okra pieces

Ghee to top each bowl

Directions

1. Put the peppers, onions and okra in the bottom of your slow cooker.

2. Put the brats on the mixture, and then add in broth. Season the ingredients with salt to your liking.

3. Put the mixture in a crockpot and cook on low for 4 to 6 hours or on high for approximately 30 minutes or instead set on simmer setting for a longer time.

4. Serve the brats with cauliflower rice.

Nutritional Information Per Serving*: Calories 222, Carbs 3.6g, Protein 18.9g, Fat 14.4g*

Egg White Vegetable Frittata

Prep Time: 10 minutes

Cook Time: 4 hours

Total Time: 4 hours 10 minutes

Serves 10

Ingredients

1/4 cup onion, diced

1 garlic clove, minced

1 1/2 cups vegetables, chopped

1/2 cup milk of your choice

1 cup low-fat cheese, shredded

2 cups egg whites

Pinch of salt & pepper

Directions

1. Using cooking spray, coat the bottom of your crockpot and set aside.

2. Then mix together all the ingredients in a medium sized bowl and stir to blend.

3. Move your mixture to the slow cooker and cover.

4. Cook on low setting until the eggs are set, or for 6 to 8 hours or on high for 3 to 4 hours.

Nutritional Information Per Serving: *Calories 92, Carbs 5g, Protein 10.5g, Fat 13.2g*

Yogurt, Kid

Prep time: 30 minutes

Cook time: 4 hours

Total time: 4 hours 30 minutes

Serves: 6

Ingredients

½ cup plain yogurt

½ gallon of whole organic milk (8 cups)

Directions

1. To make the yoghurt, first add half gallon of milk into a crockpot.

2. Then insert your thermometer into the crockpot and secure it to prevent it from slipping inside.

3. Press on the "BOIL" setting and now stir the milk so that it doesn't scald as it heats up.

4. Keep a close eye on the temperature. As soon as it reaches 200 degrees, quickly turn off the crockpot.

5. At this point, scoop any amount of milk from the crockpot and move it to a medium mixing bowl.

6. Add in ½ cup of premade yoghurt and stir to blend the mixture. Allow the milk to get to 112 degrees.

7. Once you achieve the temperatures, pour the mixture into the crockpot and whisk until well incorporated.

8. Cover the crockpot, pile some heavy clothing such as brackets and wait for approximately 4 hours.

9. Then move the yoghurt to the fridge or instead pour in a jar and store in cold setting to set.

10. In case you want a tarter taste, let the yoghurt to set for around 5 to 6 hours before you keep it chilled to set.

Calories 211, Carbs 6.5g, Protein 10.9g, Fat 11.3g

Santa Fe Omelet

Prep Time: 5 minutes

Cook Time: 3 hours

Total Time: 3 hours 5 minutes

Serves 4

Ingredients

1¼ cup Monterey Jack cheese

9 eggs, beaten

¼ cup chopped green pepper

¼ cup chopped onion

2 - Ounce can chopped green chilies

½ pound ground pork breakfast sausage browned and drained.

Salt and pepper, to taste

Optional: sour cream, salsa and green onions

Directions

1. Layer onion, sausage, green pepper, chilies and cheese in a well-greased crockpot.

2. Then cover with eggs and cover. Cook on low settings for approximately 3 to 4 hours.

3. Once cooked through, garnish as you want. Note that if using a 6-quart crockpot, you can consider doubling the recipe.

Nutritional Information Per Serving: Calories 730, Carbs 7.6g, Protein 47.8g, Fat 56.0g

Crust-less Broccoli Cheese Quiche

Prep time: 20 minutes

Cook time: 2 hours 15 minutes

Total time: 2 hours 35 minutes

Serves: 8

Ingredients

2 cups of Colby-Jack shredded cheese

1 (8-oz.) pkg. cream cheese

¼ teaspoon onion powder

¼ teaspoon pepper

¾ teaspoon salt

9 eggs

3 cups cut broccoli

Directions

1. Put a pot of boiling water on a stop-top pressure cooker and bring to a boil. Add in broccoli to the boiling water.

2. Cook for no more than 3 minutes, then drain and rinse using cold water. Set the broccoli aside.

3. Now to a large bowl, add in egg, onion powder, pepper, salt and cream cheese.

4, Beat on medium speed using a hand-held mixer until well incorporated. You may as well leave a few chunks of the cream cheese in the mixture.

5. At this point, spray your crockpot with spray and add in boiled broccoli evenly in the cooking pot.

6. Spray with half cup of cream cheese and then pour over the egg and onion powder mixture.

7. Seal the lid in place and cook for 2 ¼ hours on high setting, without opening the lid anytime during cooking.

8. As soon as the broccoli cheese quiche is cooked through, sprinkle the reserved cheese and cover. Allow the cheese to melt for approximately 10 minutes and then serve.

Nutritional Information Per Serving*: Calories 368, Carbs 3.6g, Protein 20.6g, Fat 30.1g*

Cream Spinach and Mozzarella Quiche

Prep Time: 5 Minutes

Cook Time: 2 hours 30 minutes

Total Time: 2 hours 35 minutes

Serves 4

Ingredients

11 ounces frozen creamed spinach

1 1/2 cups mozzarella cheese shredded

6 whole eggs

Directions

1. Beat eggs in a medium-sized bowl. Then add in the cream spinach and cheese and combine well.

2. Pour the mixture into a heat-safe pan that can easily fit in the slow cooker.

3. Cook on high setting for 2-2 ½ hours. Serve once the eggs are solid and you can notice the white liquid of cream and cheese.

Nutritional Information Per Serving: Calories 277, Carbs 6.3g, Protein 14.9g, Fat 29.7g

Spinach Quiche

Prep Time: 15minutes

Cook Time: 4hours on LOW

Total Time: 4 hours 15 minutes

Servings: 6

Ingredients

1 1/2 cups fresh spinach, cut up

1/2 cup onion finely diced

6 links sausage cooked, bite sized pieces

1/2 tablespoons each ground black pepper + salt

2 cups cheddar cheese, grated

1 cup milk

10 whole eggs beaten

Directions

1. In a bowl, beat the eggs well and then add in salt, cheese, milk and pepper.

2. Add onion, spinach along with the cooked links sausage.

3. At this point, line your slow cooker with a liner and coat it with pam.

4. Transfer the mixture into the slow cooker and cover. Cook on low setting for about 4 hours or so.

Nutritional Information Per Serving: *Calories 551, Carbs 7.5g, Protein 40.7g, Fat 59g*

Sausage Bake

Prep Time: 15 minutes

Cook Time: 2 to 3 hours

Total Time: 3 hours 15 minutes

Serves 4

Ingredients

1/2 pound turkey sausage, cooked and drained

1 cup mozzarella cheese, shredded

1 whole egg

3/4 cup milk whole milk preferred

1/4 teaspoon garlic powder

3/4 teaspoon baking powder

3/4 cup all-purpose flour

Directions

1. In a bowl, mix together baking powder, flour and garlic.

2. Then add in egg and milk and stir well to blend. Add in the rest of the ingredients and combine well.

3. Grease the insides of a slow cooker and pour the mixture into the cooking pot.

4. Now cook the ingredients on low setting until the mixture is done in the middle, or for 2 to 3 hours.

5. Serve the bake and enjoy.

Nutritional Information Per Serving: *Calories 258, Carbs 12g, Protein 24g, Fat 24.9g*

Bacon & Egg Casserole

Prep Time: 5 minutes

Cook Time: 2 hours 30 minutes

Total Time: 2 hours 35 minutes

Serves 4

Ingredients

6 whole eggs

1/4 teaspoon dried oregano

1/2 teaspoon ground mustard

2 cups milk

1 cup Colby and Jack cheese shredded

1 cup baking mix

1 pound bacon cooked, drained, and chopped

Directions

1. Combine all ingredients in a bowl using a whisk.

2. Transfer the mixture to a slow cooker and cover.

3. Cook on high until a knife stuck in the center comes out clean, or for about 2 ½ hours.

4. Devour!

Nutritional Information Per Serving: *Calories 862, Carbs 9g, Protein 39.4g, Fat 73.7g*

Biscuit Breakfast Casserole

Prep Time: 15 minutes

Cook Time: 1 hour 30 minutes on high

Total Time: 1 hour 45 minutes

Serves 6

Ingredients

Butter

5 oz. bacon (cooked and chopped)

1/2 cup cheddar cheese (shredded)

1/4 cup milk

4 whole eggs

7.5 oz. refrigerated biscuits (1 five count can)

Directions

1. Grease or butter the bottom and sides of a slow cooker.

2. Then layer the biscuits at the bottom of the cooking pan.

3. Then in a different bowl, mix together bacon, cheese, milks and eggs; and now pour this mixture on the biscuits.

4. Cover and cook on high until the sides of the slow cooker show light brown biscuits, or for about 1 hour 30 minutes.

Nutritional Information Per Serving: *Calories 313, Carbs 9.2g, Protein 13.5g, Fat 20.6g*

Frittata with Artichoke Hearts, Red Pepper, and Feta

Prep Time: 30 minutes

Cook Time: 2-3 hours

Total Time: 2 1/2 - 3 1/2 hours

Serves 6-8

Ingredients

4 oz. crumbled Feta cheese

8 eggs, completely combined yolks and whites

1/4 cup green onions, sliced

1 jar (12 oz.) roasted red peppers, cut into small pieces

1 can (14 oz.) artichoke hearts, cut into small pieces

Black pepper, freshly ground

1 teaspoon Spike Seasoning

2 tablespoons chopped parsley, optional

Directions

1. In a colander that is put in a sink, add in the artichokes from the can and allow them to drain fully.

2. Meanwhile, crumble the feta cheese and start slicing the onions. Then coat your crockpot with cooking spray. Go for the non-stick spray of course!

3. Once completely drain, remove the artichokes from the colander and put them on a cutting board. To the colander, pour the roasted red peppers to drain as well.

4. Now cut the artichokes into quarters or other small pieces you can manage. Add the hearts to the bottom of a crockpot insert. (You should use a 5 or 6 quart slow cooker for this).

5. Pour the drained red peppers from the colander to the cutting board. Then cut them into half-inch squares and add them to the crockpot. Top the mixture with the green onions.

6. Now beat the eggs well to fully incorporate eggs yolks and egg whites. Pour the whisked eggs over the veggies in the crockpot.

7. Stir the mixture using a fork to well distribute the green onions, red pepper pieces and the sliced artichoke hearts.

8. At this point, sprinkle the cheese over the ingredients and then season with black pepper and the spike seasoning.

9. Cook the frittata mixture on low setting until the eggs are firm and the feta has melted, or for about 2 to 3 hours depending on the crockpot you have. (Ninja cookers are somehow hotter!)

10. Now cut the frittata into various portions while still in the crockpot. Serve it hot while garnished with chopped parsley if you like.

Nutritional Information Per Serving: *Calories 188, Carbs 6.4g, Protein 12g, Fat 16.8g*

Pizza Casserole

Prep Time: 15 minutes

Cook Time: 2 hours

Total Time: 2 hours 15 minutes

Serves 6

Ingredients

2 cups shredded mozzarella cheese

1 (8-oz) package baby bella mushrooms

1 medium onion

1 large green pepper

1 (14-oz) jar pizza sauce

1 lb. ground beef

Pepperoni slices

Directions

1. First dice the onion, green pepper and the mushrooms. Then add the diced vegetables to a pan along with the ground beef.

2. Cook the mixture in the pan until the vegetables are tender and the beef has browned.

3. Drain and then layer the mixture in a slow cooker along with pepperoni, cheese and the pizza sauce. Repeat the layers as you desire.

4. Cook the casserole mixture on low setting until cooked through and the cheese has melted, or for approximately 2 hours.

Nutritional Information Per Serving: *Calories 303, Carbs 10g, Protein 16.9g, Fat 26.5g*

Lunch Recipes

Shredded Chicken

Prep Time: 5 minutes

Cook Time: 3 hours 30 minutes

Total Time: 3 hours 35 minutes

Servings: 8 cups

Ingredients

1/2 cup low sodium chicken broth

1/2 ounce garlic powder

1/2 ounce black pepper

1 ounce kosher salt

3 pounds boneless skinless chicken breasts

Directions

1. Add in chicken broth in a crockpot and then add in the chicken. Season the chicken with garlic powder, pepper and salt. (Broth is not required if you're using a frozen meat).

2. Cook the chicken on high heat for approximately 4 hours or on low heat for 5 hours.

3. Then shred the cooked chicken using two forks. Return the shredded meat to the crockpot and cook for another 30

minutes or so on low heat setting to help moisten and tenderize the chicken. This also adds flavor.

4. At this point, divide the chicken into 2 cups or other 2 equal portions based on your preference.

5. Put the chicken in freezer bags and keep it frozen for not more than 4 months.

6. To serve, add thawed chicken to soups, casseroles and sandwiches.

Nutritional Information Per Serving: *Calories 208, Carb 0.4g, Protein 4.5g, Fat 38.6g*

Salsa Chicken

Prep Time 5 minutes

Cook Time 2 hours 15 minutes

Total Time 2 hours 20 minutes

Serves 6

Ingredients

1 1/2 cups shredded cheese Kraft Mexican blend

1 1/2 cups fresh salsa

1 1/2 lb. chicken breasts boneless, skinless

Directions

1. Using olive oil, lightly grease a slow cooker then add in whole chicken breasts.

2. Add salsa over the meat and now cook on high heat for approximately 2 hours.

3. Meanwhile, preheat your oven to 425 degrees F. Put the meat in a lightly coated baking dish and cover using the salsa from the slow cooker. Drain all the fluids.

4. Top the chicken with cheese and bake for approximately 15 minutes, or until the cheese and the sauce starts to bubble.

5. Now you can serve garnished with full fat sour cream or fresh cilantro.

Nutritional Information Per Serving*: Calories 314, Carbs 4.8g, Protein 18.6g, Fat 31.2g*

Italian Beef

Prep Time: 20 minutes

Cook Time: 10 hours

Total Time: 10 hours 20 minutes

Serves 6

Ingredients

1 1/2 cups beef broth

1 large onion sliced

1 tablespoon Italian Seasoning

1 boneless beef chuck roast 3-1/2 to 4 pounds

1 jar 12 ounces whole pepperoncini with the liquid

Directions

1. Put the beef chuck roast in a freezer bag and add in the pepperoncini. Add in the onion along with Italian seasoning and freeze the mixture.

2. Once ready to cook beef, thaw the meat in the fridge, preferably overnight. Put in a crockpot and add in broth.

4. Cover the ingredients and cook on low setting for about 10 hours.

5. As soon as the roast is tender, just shred it using two forks. Serve the beef, onions and peppers with a slotted spoon and enjoy.

Nutritional Information Per Serving: Calories 221, Cars 5g, Protein 21g, Fat 28.3g

5-Ingredient Garlic Balsamic Chicken

Prep Time: 15 minutes

Cook Time: 3 to 4 hours

Total Time: 4 hours 15 minutes

Serves 5 to 8

Ingredients

3 ½ pounds bone-in, skin-on chicken breasts

1 ounce kosher salt

2 tablespoons olive oil

¼ cup balsamic vinegar

2 medium garlic cloves, minced or finely grated

Directions

1. In a crockpot, whisk together olive oil, balsamic vinegar, garlic and salt.

2. Then add in the chicken and toss to coat. Cover the chicken and cook on high heat for 3 to 4 hours or on low heat for 5 to 6 hours.

3. As soon as the chicken is cooked through, remove it from the crockpot, skin it if you like it and then serve.

4. In case you want the skin intact, put the meat on a sheet pan and broil on high heat until it's crispy, or for about 5 to 8 minutes.

5. Strain any of the juices from crockpot and serve the dish preferably warm.

Nutritional Information Per Serving: *Calories 232, Carbs 7.4g, Protein 24.6g, Fat 27g*

Steak Fajitas

Prep Time: 10 minutes

Cook Time: 3 hours

Total Time: 3 hours 10 minutes

Serves 6

Ingredients

2 tablespoons fajita seasoning

15 ounces salsa or diced tomatoes

1 onion, sliced

1-2 bell peppers, sliced

2 lbs. beef, sliced

Directions

1. To a crockpot, add in all the ingredients in whichever order then stir to blend well.

2. Cook the ingredients on high for 2 to 3 hours or at low heat for about 4 to 6 hours.

3. Then remove from the slow cooker and serve.

Nutritional Information Per Serving: *Calories 242, Carbs 7.7g, Protein 33.8g, Fat 8.1g*

Southern Roast

Prep Time: 5 minutes

Cook Time: 10 hours

Total Time: 10 hours 5 minutes

Serves 6

Ingredients

1 stick of butter 1/2 cup

5-6 Pepperoncino peppers

1 packet of au jus mix

1 packet of Ranch Seasoning mix or homemade mix

3-5 lb. chuck roast

Directions

1. Put the chuck roast in a crockpot and sprinkle with the seasoning mix. Put pepperoncino on the chuck roast with the stick of butter.

2. Cover the contents in the crockpot and cook on low setting for approximately 10 hours.

3. Once cooked through, remove the roast from the crockpot and serve it.

Nutritional Information Per Serving: *Calories 645, Carbs 7g, Protein 42.9g, Fat 57.6g*

Simple Poached Salmon

Prep Time: 15 minutes

Cook Time: 20 minutes

Total Time: 35 minutes

Serves 4

Ingredients

4 (6-ounce) salmon fillets

1/2 ounce salt

1 sprig dill

1 lemon slice

1 yellow onion slice

1/2 cup dry white wine

1 cup water

Directions

1. Mix together wine and water in a crockpot. Then heat the mixture on high for about 20 to 30 minutes.

2. Now add in the salmon, salt, dill, lemon and onion.

3. Cover the mixture and cook on high setting for approximately 20 minutes.

4. As soon as the salmon is cooked through and is opaque, remove from the slow cooker and taste.

5. Serve it whether hot or cold as per your liking.

Nutritional Information Per Serving: *Calories 313, Carbs 3.6g, Protein 28.4g, Fat 25.2g*

Taco Chicken

Prep Time: 15 minutes

Cook Time: 4 hours

Total Time: 4 hours 15 minutes

Serves 8

Ingredients

2 – 16 ounce jars salsa Verde

2 1/2 pounds boneless skinless chicken breasts

Directions

1. Set a crockpot to low setting, and then pour a jar of salsa Verde in the bottom.

2. Add in chicken breasts and season with some salt over the top. Then pour in the rest of salsa Verde over the meat.

3. Cover the mixture and cook on high for 3 to 4 hours or on low setting for 6 to 8 hours.

4. As soon as the chicken is cooked through, remove it from the stock.

5. Shred the chicken using two forks and then return the shredded meat back into the stock.

6. Turn the crockpot on warm setting until you'll ready to serve.

Nutritional Information Per Serving: *Calories 161, Carbs 0g, Protein 3g, Fat 30g*

Garlic Beef Roast

Prep Time 5 minutes

Cook Time 10 hours

Total Time 10 hours 5 minutes

Serves 6

Ingredients

Salt

Pepper

1 stick of butter

2 tablespoon minced garlic

3-5 lb. beef roast

Directions

1. Put the beef roast in a crockpot and generously season with garlic.

2. Season with pepper and salt then add stick of butter on top. Cover the crockpot and cook on low heat for about 10 hours.

3. Then remove from the cooking pot and enjoy.

Nutritional Information Per Serving: *Calories 693, Carbs 0.9g, Protein 80g, Fat 41g*

Cheddar Cream of Mushroom Chicken

Prep Time: 15 minutes

Cook Time: 30 minutes

Total Time: 45 minutes

Serves 4

Ingredients

2 boneless skinless chicken breasts

1 can of French's cheddar French fried onions

1 can of family size cream of mushroom soup

Directions

1. Preheat your crockpot to oven bake at about 275 degrees F.

2. Then put the chicken breasts into the bottom of the slow cooker and spread it evenly apart.

3. Pour the cream of mushroom soup on the meat and let it cook for a few hours.

4. Approximately 30 minutes before cooking is over, sprinkle the tops of the chicken breasts with fried onions and continue to cook until cooked through.

5. Serve the cheddar cream of mushroom chicken with veggies and enjoy.

Nutritional Information Per Serving: *Calories 335, Carbs 6.4g, protein 22.8g, Fat 39.5g*

Hawaiian Pulled Pork

Total Time: 10 minutes

Prep Time: 2 minutes

Cook Time: 8 minutes

Serves 6

Ingredients:

2 tablespoons pink Hawaiian salt

1 1/2 tablespoons olive oil

3 lbs. boneless pork butt/shoulder

Directions

1. Stab the pork butt or shoulder on all sides about 3 to 4 times, and then coat it with olive oil.

2. Sprinkle each side of the pork with salt and put the meat in a crockpot.

3. Cover and cook on low for approximately 7 hours, or until cooked through.

4. Then remove from the crockpot and shred the pork using 2 forks. Return it back to the crockpot and cook for another 1 hour.

Nutritional Information Per Serving: *Calories: 452, Carbs 0g, Protein: 39.5g, Fat: 31.4g*

Buffalo Chicken

Prep Time: 15 minutes

Cook Time: 6 hours on LOW

Total Time: 6 hours 15 minutes

Servings: 6

Ingredients

3 tablespoons butter

1/2 packets hidden valley ranch

1 bottles hot sauce

6 chicken breasts

Directions

1. Add in the chicken in a crockpot and then pour hot sauce over the meat. Season the chicken with the ranch.

2. Cover the mixture and now cook on low setting for approximately 6 hours.

3. Then shred the chicken, add in butter and cook on how setting for another 1 hour.

Nutritional Information Per Serving: *Calories 297.0, Carbs 2.0g, Fats 8.0g, Protein 52.0g*

Caesar Pork Chops

Prep Time 5 minutes

Cook Time 8 hours

Total Time 8 hours 5 minutes

Serves 4

Ingredients

2 cups fresh green beans

4-6 pork chops

10 ounce Caesar dressing

Salt and pepper

Directions

1. First season the pork chops with salt and pepper. Put the pork in a freezer-friendly bag and keep frozen.

2. Once ready to cook, just thaw in the fridge for a few hours.

3. Then add to the crockpot and cook on low setting for about 6 to 8 hours.

4. Serve and enjoy.

Nutritional Information Per Serving: *Calories 811, Carbs 5.6g, Protein 52.7g, Fat 63g*

Lemon Chicken

Prep Time: 5 minutes

Cook Time: 4 hours

Total Time: 4 hours 5 minutes

Serves: 4

Ingredients

2 lemons

1 0.7 ounce envelope Italian salad dressing mix

4 boneless, skinless chicken breasts

2 tablespoons butter

Directions

1. Add butter to a slow cooker and then add in the meat.

2. Add in lemon juice over the meat and season with the salad dressing mix.

3. Cook the chicken on low setting for approximately 4 hours.

Nutritional Information Per Serving: *Calories: 195, Carbs 5g, Protein 8g, Fat 24g*

Balsamic Glazed Short Ribs

Prep Time: 15 minutes

Cook Time: 6 hours

Total Time: 6 hours 15 minutes

Serves 8

Ingredients

1 teaspoon of ground rosemary

2 large cloves of garlic

1/4 cup balsamic vinegar

1/2 cup dry red wine or broth

Salt and pepper

4 ribs bone in beef short ribs

1 tablespoon of olive oil

Directions

1. Over medium-high heat, heat some oil in a heavy skillet until hot enough.

2. Meanwhile, you can put the short-ribs in the microwave for 1-2 minutes to thaw especially if from the fridge- cold ribs may stick to the pan.

3. You may also need to trim some fat from the ribs before browning. Season the short ribs with some pepper and salt.

4. Now brown the ribs on all sides, dealing with a few of them at a time. Ensure that you brown the fatty parts too.

5. Move the browned short ribs to the crockpot and add the rest of the ingredients.

6. Cover and cook on low until they are fork tender, or about 6 hours. Turn them half-way through for uniform cooking.

7. Once cooked through, turn the ribs and dip them in the slow cooker before serving.

8. Top with vegetables or a green salad.

Nutritional Information Per Serving*: Calories 391, Carbs 6.5g, Protein 42g, Fat 33.4g*

Chicken Tacos

Prep Time 5 minutes

Cook Time 8 hours

Total Time 8 hours 5 minutes

Serves 6

Ingredients

1 onion, diced

1 15 ounce can of diced tomatoes

1 packet of taco seasoning

3-4 boneless skinless chicken breasts

Tortillas: sour cream, shredded cheese, lettuce

Directions

1. Put the skinless meat in the bottom of a crockpot and sprinkle with the taco packet.

2. Pour tomatoes on top, but leave some liquid in the can. Add in diced onion on the tomato and chicken mixture and cover the slow cooker.

3. Cook on low setting for approximately 8 to 10 hours. As soon as the chicken is cooked through, shred it and stir to blend.

4. Cook for another 10 minutes and then serve with favorite toppings.

Nutritional Information Per Serving: Calories 226, Carbs 3g, Protein 22.7g, Fat 16.4g

Dinner Recipes

Crock-Pot Mississippi Roast

Prep Time: 20minutes

Cook Time: 8 hours on LOW

Serves 6

Ingredients

4 - 8 jarred pepperoncini peppers whole

1/2 cup salted butter or less if the roast has extra fat

1 cup bistro au jus gravy or any canned or jarred brown gravy

1 packet of ranch dressing mix

1 large yellow onion, sectioned

Salt and pepper to taste

2 pounds beef chuck roast

2 - 3 tablespoons olive oil, optional

Directions

1. Season both sides of the beef with pepper and salt and put in the bottom of a large crockpot. To get a darker roast, consider searing the meat in a frying pan for a couple of minutes.

2. Surround the beef chuck roast with onions to help have a roast that is lying as flat as possible in the bottom of a slow cooker.

3. Pour a cup of homemade gravy or the au jus gravy over the meat and sprinkle with the dressing mix. The gravy helps the dressing stick well to the roast.

4. Cut the stick butter into chunks and then put the cut butter on the roast. Spread them all along the meat.

5. Now layer a few pepperoncini peppers on the beef and cover the crockpot. Cook the mixture on low setting until the roast reaches a temperature of 145 degrees, or for approximately 8 hours.

6. Remove the pepperoncini a few minutes before serving, or eat them too if you want.

7. Shred the cooked beef with forks and serve topped with cooking juices from the crockpot as gravy.

Nutritional Information Per Serving: *Calories: 608, Carbs: 8g, Protein: 30g, Fat: 49g*

Beef Chuck Pot Roast

Preparation: 5 minutes

Cooking: 3-5 hours

Total Time: 5 hours

Servings: 10

Ingredients

1 onion soup dry mix (use 1 packet)

1 can cream of celery soup or cream of mushroom soup

4 lbs. beef for roasting

Directions

1. Begin by stabbing the meat in a few places using a fork or knife, and place in crock pot with side with the fatty side facing up.

2. Add dry onion soup to the sides ad on top followed with celery soup or the can of mushroom over the roast.

3. Spread it on top a little and now cover the slow cooker and turn it on!

4. At this point, cook for 3 hours on high or 5 hours set on low heat setting.

5. If need be, set the slow cooker on low and allow the roast in- in the morning to prepare for an evening meal.

Nutritional Information Per Serving: *Calories 280, Carbs 2.5g, Protein 22g, Fat 13.2g*

Swiss Steak

Prep Time: 10 min

Cook Time: 6 hours

Total Time: 6 hours 10 minutes

Serves 6

Ingredients

2 cans 8-ounces tomato sauce

1 celery rib, cut into 1/2-inch slices

1 medium onion, cut into 1/4-inch slices

1-1/2 pounds beef round steak, cut into six pieces

1/4 ounce pepper

1/2 ounce salt

2 tablespoons all-purpose flour

Directions

1. Mix the flour, pepper and salt in a large re-sealable bag.

2. Add in the steak, seal the plastic bag and shake well to coat.

3. Put the onion in a greased crockpot and top with tomato sauce, celery and the steak.

4. Cover the contents and cook on low heat until the meat is done or for about 6 to 8 hours.

Nutritional Information Per Serving: *Calories 171, Carb 6g, Project 4g, Fat 27g*

Garlic Chicken Drumsticks

Prep Time 10 minutes

Cook Time 8 hours

Total Time 8 hours 10 minutes

Serves 4

Ingredients

1 cup chicken broth

6 whole garlic cloves

1 ounce ground paprika

1/4 cup olive oil

8 fresh chicken legs 2 per person

1 cup fresh onion sliced thin

Directions

1. Add all ingredients, apart from the broth, to a freezer-friendly bag.

2. Combine well until incorporated, and then keep frozen. When ready to cook, thaw overnight in the fridge.

3. Add to a crockpot along with broth and cook on low setting for approximately 6 to 8 hours.

4. If you want, move to a baking dish and broil for approximately 4 minutes on high seat setting to help crisp the skin.

Nutritional Information Per Serving: *Calories 631, Carbs 8g, Protein 51.6g, Fat 54.2g*

Easy Chili Verde

Prep Time: 10 minutes

Cook Time: 5 hours

Total Time: 5 hours 10 minutes

Serves 12

Ingredients

1/2 ounce salt

1 4-ounce can chopped green chilies

1 cup salsa Verde

3 10-ounce cans green enchilada sauce

1 boneless pork shoulder roast, cut into 1-inch pieces

Sour cream, optional

Directions

1. Mix together green chiles, salsa Verde, enchilada sauce, pork and salt in a crockpot.

2. Cook the mixture on low setting until the pork is tender, or for about 5 to 6 hours.

3. Top the chili with sour cream and enjoy.

Nutritional Information Per Serving: Calories 287, Carbs 5g, Protein 27g, Fat 17g

Java Roast Beef

Prep Time: 10 min

Cook Time: 8 hours

Total Time: 8 hours 10 minutes

Serves 12

Ingredients

1/4 cup cold water

2 tablespoons cornstarch

1 1/2 cups strong brewed coffee

1 boneless beef chuck roast

3/4 ounce pepper

1 1/2 ounces salt

5 garlic cloves, minced

Directions

1. Combine salt, garlic and pepper then tub this seasoning over the beef.

2. Move to a crockpot and now pour in coffee around the beef. Cook while covered until the beef is tender, or on low for 8 to 10 hours.

3. Move the cooked meat to a serving plate and keep it warm.

4. Meanwhile, move the cooking juices to a saucepan skim fat off and then bring the stock to a boil.

5. Combine water and cornstarch in a separate bowl until smooth, and then stir the thickener into the cooking stock.

6. Let boil and then cook until thickened, or for about 1 to 2 minutes. Serve the sauce with the roast beef.

Nutritional Information Per Serving: *Calories 199, Carbs 2g, Protein 22g, Fat 11g*

Kalua Pig

Prep: 15 minutes

Cook: 12 hours

Total: 12 hours, 15 minutes

Serves 8

Ingredients

5 peeled garlic cloves

1½ tablespoons of sea salt

5 pound Boston butt roast bone-in or out

3 slices of bacon

Directions

1. Line a crockpot with the bacon slices. If you want it, you can first remove the skin from the bacon with a knife.

2. Season with sea salt and now cut a few slits into the pork. Tuck in a few garlic cloves too, and then salt the meat allover.

3. Put the pork butt roast on top of the sliced bacon in a crockpot, with skin side facing up.

4. Cover and cook the butt roast on low setting for approximately 16 hours, without adding any liquid in. (take note that newer crockpots may require as little as 9 to 12 hours on low heat setting).

5. As soon as the pork is cooked through, remove from the crockpot and use 2 forks to shred it.

6. Taste the seasoning and adjust the flavor using the liquid that accumulate on the bottom of cooking pot.

7. Enjoy the kalua pig!

Nutritional Information Per Serving: Calories 621, Carbs 0.7g, Protein 50g, Fat 60.6g

3 Ingredient Pork Dinner

Prep Time: 15 minutes

Cook Time: 4 to 5 hours

Total Time: 5 hours 15 minutes

Serves 6

Ingredients

2-3 pounds of pork roast

1 packet of onion soup mix

1 can of dr. pepper

Directions

1. First cut the pork roast into various sections to help fit in the slow cooker.

2. Then flip the cut pieces in the onion soup mix to coat them well.

3. Now layer the coated pork pieces into the slow cooker and then pour in the Dr. Pepper over the chunks till almost covered.

4. At this point, cook the pork on high until cooked through, or for about 4 to 5 hours.

5. Drain off any accumulated fluid in the cooker, shred the cooked pork. Serve!

Nutritional Information Per Serving: *Calories 385, Carbs 4.9g, Protein 20.6g, Fat 46.7g*

Rump Roast with Onions

Prep Time: 5 minutes

Cook Time: 8 hours

Total Time: 8 hours 5 minutes

Serves 4-6

Ingredients

1/2 cup beef broth

1 ounce minced garlic

1 1/2 ounces salt

2 ounces black pepper

2 onions thinly sliced

3 - 4 lb. rump roast

Directions

1. Put the roast in a slow cooker and spread the onions on the meat.

2. Combine beef broth, garlic, salt and pepper in a small bowl.

3. Pour this mixture over the top of the roast and seal the lid in place.

4. Now cook on low heat setting for about 8 to 10 hours.

Nutritional Information Per Serving: *Calories 474, Carbs 6g, Protein 54.6g, Fat 34.7g*

Easy Turkey Breast

Prep Time: 15 minutes

Cook Time: 6 hours

Total Time: 6 to 7 hours

Serves 10

Ingredients

3 tablespoons butter

1 packet dry onion soup mix

1 turkey breast (bone in) about 6 pounds

Directions

1. First coat the inside of your slow cooker with spray and add in the turkey, breast side facing up.

2. Coat the breast generously with the dry onion soup mix.

3. Then cut butter into 3 equal portions and put on top of the seasoned turkey breast.

4. Cook the meat on low setting until it reaches temperatures of 175 degrees F, or for approximately 6 to 7 hours.

Nutritional Information Per Serving: *Calories 397, Carbs 2.5g, Protein 29.9g, Fat 39.4g*

Chicken Stroganoff

Prep time: 10 minutes

Cook Time: 5 hours

Total Time: 5 hours 10 minutes

Serves: 4

Ingredients

1 (10.75 ounce) can-condensed cream, chicken soup

1 (8 ounce) package of cream cheese

1 (7 ounce) package of dry Italian style salad dressing mixture

1/8 cup of margarine

4 skinless, boneless chicken breasts halves (cubed)

Directions

1. Place the chicken, dressing and margarine into a Crock Pot and mix together.

2. Cook on low heat for 6 hours.

3. Then add in the cream cheese, the soup and combine together.

4. Finally, cook on high heat for an extra ½ hour or until it is warm and heated through.

Nutritional Information Per Serving: *Calories 456, Carbs 9.5g, Protein 33.4g, Fat 31g*

Montreal Chuck Roast

Prep Time: 5 minutes

Cook Time: 8 hours

Total Time: 8 hours 5 minutes

Serves 4

Ingredients

1 tablespoon minced onion

2 tablespoons McCormick Montreal steak seasoning

1 cup beef broth

3-5 lb. chuck roast

Directions

1. Put the chuck roast in a crockpot, add in broth and season with the steak seasoning.

2. Add a lid and cook on low heat for around 8 hours. Then remove the cover and serve the chuck roast.

Nutritional Information Per Serving: *Calories 628, Carbs 3g, Protein 64.5g, Fat 56.3g*

Homemade Italian Beef

Prep Time 15minutes

Cook Time: 6 hours on LOW

Servings: 12

Ingredients

8 ounces Italian style sandwich mix peppers

28 ounces beef broth

16 ounces pepperoncini peppers

1 ounce Italian dressing dry mix

3 pounds beef roast

Directions

1. Add the beef roast, peppers, beef broth and dressing mix in a large slow cooker.

2. Cover the mixture and cook on low until the beef roast is tender and can easily be shredded using a fork, or for approximately 6 hours.

3. Then remove the cooked beef from the crockpot and put in a rimmed baking sheet.

4. Using a fork, shred the beef and discard any bones if present; and now return it into the crockpot along with the coking liquids.

5. Cook the meat on high setting for another 1 hour. At this point, serve the meat topped with provolone cheese if you like.

Nutritional Information Per Serving: *Calories: 341, Carbs: 5g, Protein: 52g, Fat: 10g*

Crust-less Pizza

Prep Time 10 minutes

Cook Time 4 hours

Total Time 4 hours 10 minutes

Serves 4

Ingredients

5-6 slices mozzarella cheese or provolone cheese

1 1/2 cups pizza sauce or marinara sauce

2 cups mozzarella cheese

2 lbs. ground beef browned

Toppings: mushrooms, pepperoni and peppers

Directions

1. Coat a slow cooker with cooking spray and then add in 2 cups of mozzarella cheese along with browned ground beef.

2. Stir to incorporate and then spread across the bottom of the cooking pan.

3. Top the ingredients with the pizza sauce evenly, and with the provolone cheese on top.

3. Top with peppers, mushrooms or other preferred toppings of choice. Cook on high for 2 hours or on low heat for approximately 4 hours.

4. Garnish with parmesan and enjoy.

Nutritional Information Per Serving: *Calories 711, Carbs 9.8g, Protein 71.3g, Fat 52.5g*

Chicken Enchilada Dip

Prep Time: 0 hours 20 minutes

Cook Time: 1 hour

Total Time: 1 hour 20 minutes

Serves 8

Ingredients

1 jalapeño, sliced

8 ounce cream cheese, softened

2 cup pepper jack, grated

1 15-oz. can enchilada sauce

1 rotisserie chicken, shredded

1 tablespoon Taco Seasoning

Directions

1. Mix together chicken, jalapeno, cream cheese, pepper jack, enchilada sauce and taco seasonings in a crockpot.

2. Cover the mixture and cook on high setting for about 1 hour.

3. Stir the mixture until creamy and then cook for another 30 to 60 minutes while covered.

4. Serve and enjoy.

Nutritional Information Per Serving: Calories 167, Carbs 6.2g, Protein 15.3g, Fat 9.1g

Whole Chicken

Prep Time 5 minutes

Cook Time 8 hours

Total Time 8 hours 5 minutes

Serves 8

Ingredients

Salt and pepper

3-4 tablespoon olive oil

5-7 lb. whole chicken rinsed and dry

Directions

1. Put the whole chicken in the slow cooker. Then rub generously with some oil and season with some pepper and salt.

2. Cover and cook in the slow cooker for at least 8 hours. Serve and enjoy.

Nutritional Information Per Serving: Calories 437, Carbs 0g, Protein 59.1g, Fat 25.9g

Chicken Taco Soup

Prep time: 15 minutes

Cook time: 6 hours

Total time: 6 hours

Serves 4

Ingredients

4 cups chicken broth

2 (10-oz) cans diced tomatoes and green chiles

3 tablespoon southwestern seasoning

1 (1-oz) package Ranch Seasoning and Salad Dressing Mix

2 (8-oz) packages cream cheese

2 lb. boneless skinless chicken breasts

Directions

1. Put all the ingredients in a crockpot.

2. Cover them and now cook on low settings for about 6 to 8 hours.

3. Then remove the chicken from the crockpot and shred it using two forks.

4. Now return the chicken to the crockpot and stir. Serve the chicken taco soup with sour cream, cilantro and cheese.

Nutritional Information Per Serving: Calories 86, Carbs 1.9g, Protein 7.6g, Fat 5.2g

Snacks and Desserts

Easy Seasoned Pecans

Total: 33 minutes

Prep: 3 minutes

Cook: 30 minutes

Serves 16

Ingredients

1 teaspoon seasoning blend

4 cups pecans (halves)

5 tablespoons plus 1 teaspoon butter (melted)

Directions

1. Get the required ingredients ready and then mix them well in the cooking pot of a crockpot.

2. Cover the mixture and then cook on high setting for around 15 minutes.

3. Then set the crockpot to low heat and now cook for another 2 hours, while uncovered. Remember to stir the ingredients a few times as cooking progresses.

4. Once cooked through, serve the pecans when ready.

Nutritional Information Per Serving: *Calories 684.1, Carbs 13.7g, Protein 9.1g, Fat 71.3g*

Peach Cobbler

Prep Time: 15 minutes

Cook Time: 2 hours

Total Time: 2 hours 15 minutes

Serves 8

Ingredients

1/2 cup butter (1 stick), softened

1 white cake mix, unprepared

6 large peaches, peeled and sliced

Directions

1. Put the sliced fruit in the bottom of a crockpot.

2. Mix together butter with the unprepared cake mix in a medium bowl. Just cut butter into the cake mix until crumbly using a potato smasher, fork or a pastry blender if you have one.

3. Then sprinkle the mixture over the sliced fruit in the crockpot.

4. Put dish towel or paper towels on the crockpot and seal it in place. Cook the mixture on high setting for 2 to 3 hours or on low for approximately 4 hours.

5. Serve the peach cobbler with vanilla ice cream if you like.

Nutritional Information Per Serving: Calories 186, Carbs 7.8g, Protein 1.8g, Fat 13g

Ranch Mushrooms

Prep Time: 15 minutes

Cook Time: 3 hours

Total Time: 3 to 4 hours

Serves 6

Ingredients

1 envelope Ranch salad dressing mix

1/2 cup butter, melted

1 pound fresh raw mushrooms

Directions

1. Put cleaned whole mushroom in a slow cooker.

2. Mix together ranch salad dressing mix with melted butter, and drizzle this mixture over the whole mushrooms.

3. Now cover and cook on low setting for 3 to 4 hours. Remember to stir after 1 hour to coat the mushroom the ingredients.

4. As soon as the mushrooms are cooked through, serve while hot.

Nutritional Information Per Serving: Calories 279, Carb 4.2g, Protein 3g, Fat 28.9g

Sweet Kielbasa

Prep Time: 10 minutes

Cook Time: 6 hours on LOW

Total Time: 6 hours and 10 minutes

Servings 32

Ingredients

2 cloves garlic minced

2 tablespoons prepared Dijon mustard

3/4 cup brown sugar packed

1 cup unsweetened apple sauce

2 pounds kielbasa sausage sliced into bite sized pieces

Directions

1. Add the above ingredients to a large crockpot and stir to mix.

2. Cover the crockpot and cook on low settings for approximately 6 hours.

3. Stir the mixture and now set the crockpot to "Warm" mode to keep the kielbasa warm before serving.

Nutritional Information Per Serving: Calories: 120, Carbs 8g, Protein 3g, Fat: 8g

Irish Cream Coffee

Prep Time: 5 minutes

Cook Time: 90 minutes on HIGH

Total: 1 hour 35 minutes

Servings 4

Ingredients

1 tablespoons cocoa powder, unsweetened

1/3 cup heavy whipping cream

1/2 cup Irish cream

3 cups strong brewed black coffee

Optional:

Chocolate shavings or sprinkles, optional

Whipped cream optional

Sweetener, optional

Directions

1. Add whipping cream, Irish cream, cocoa powder and coffee to a slow cooker and stir to mix. You can add a Keto-friendly sweetener if you like it.

2. Cover the mixture and cook on low settings for approximately 3 hours or on high for around 1 hour 30 minutes.

3. Ladle the ready coffee in mugs and top with chocolate shavings and whipped cream if you like it. If using a 6 quart slow cooker, consider doubling the recipe for more cream coffee.

Nutritional Information Per Serving: *Calories: 161, Carbs: 4g, Protein: 6g, Fat: 11g*

Crockpot Brussels Sprouts

Prep Time 10 minutes

Cook Time 2 hours on high

Total Time: 2 hours 10 minutes

Serves 6

Ingredients

1 tablespoon Dijon mustard

3 tablespoons butter

1 pound Brussels sprouts

Pepper to taste

Salt to taste

Directions

1. Prepare the Brussels sprouts: wash them and trim the ends of. Then add them to a large crockpot.

2. Add in salt, Dijon mustard and pepper then toss to coats with the Brussels. Top with 3 tablespoons of butter.

3. Cover the ingredients and cook on high settings for around 2 hours or so.

Nutritional Information Per Serving: *Calories: 88, Carbs: 5g, Protein: 8g, Fat: 16g*

Brownie Pudding

Prep Time: 15 minutes

Cook Time: 2 hours

Total Time: 2 hours 15 minutes

Serves 10

Ingredients

1 3.4 ounce box instant chocolate

3 tablespoons water

1/2 cup vegetable oil

2 large eggs water and oil

1 (15 ounce) box Brownie Mix see note

Ice cream or whipped cream

2 cups milk regular or non-fat

Directions

1. Coat a 6 quart crockpot with spray. Meanwhile, start making the brownie mix by combining it with oil, eggs and water, or as instructed on the packaging.

2. Pour the mixture into the crockpot.

3. In medium bowl, whisk together milk and pudding mix until well blended. Pour the mixture over the prepared brownie mix in the slow cooker.

4. Cover the slow cooker using paper towel and put it on top. Cook the ingredients on high settings for around 2 to 3 hours.

5. Keep watch on the edges for signs of doneness, should be somehow dry. Be aware that a little amount of the pudding with stay somehow wet until cooked through, or after hours or so. However, don't overcook the brownie.

6. Serve the brownie pudding with whipped cream or ice cream. Store any remainder in an airtight container in the fridge for not more than 3 days.

Nutritional Information Per Serving*: Calories 138, Carbs 2g, Protein 3g, Fat 13g*

Steak Bites

Prep Time 10 minutes

Cook Time 8 hours

Total Time 8 hours 10 minutes

Serves 4

Ingredients

4 tablespoons thinly sliced butter

1/2 ounce black pepper

1/2 ounce salt

1 ounce garlic powder

1 tablespoon minced onion

1/2 cup beef broth

3-4 lb. round steak

Directions

1. Cut the steak into cubes and add to the slow cooker.

2. Then gently pour the broth over the cubed steak and sprinkle with garlic, minced onion, pepper and salt.

3. Layer some sliced butter on top and seal the lid in place. Cook the ingredients on high setting for 3 to 4 hours or on low heat for 6 to 8 hours.

4. Then open the crockpot and serve.

Nutritional Information Per Serving: *Calories 779, Carbs 7g, Protein 79g, Fat 56.8g*

Dulce de Leche

Prep Time: 15 minutes

Cook Time: 10 hours on LOW

Total Time: 10 hours 15 minutes

Serves 24 ounces (8 servings)

Ingredients

Water

3-8 ounce jars with rings and lids or 4-6 ounce jars

2 cans 14 ounces each condensed milk, unsweetened

Directions

1. Divide the milk into three or four jars, those that can easily fit in your slow cooker with 1 to 2 inches of water covering them.

2. Seal the jars using lids and clean rings, and then put them in the crockpot. ensuring that they don't touch.

3. Now fill the slow cooker with water to reach about 1 to 2 inches above the jars. Then cover the crockpot.

4. Cook the contents on low settings for approximately 10 hours. Once cooked through, remove the jars from the crockpot with tongs.

5. Put the jars on a kitchen counter and let cool to room temperature. Then keep them chilled in the fridge and until ready to serve.

6. Store any remaining dulce de leche for up to a month in the refrigerator. In case you note some rust spots on the rings, wipe them using kitchen towel.

Nutritional Information Per Serving: *Calories 61, Carbs 4g, Protein 5.1g, Fat 6.2g*

Crock Pot Candy

Prep Time: 15 minutes

Cook Time: 1-2 hours

Total Time: 2 hours

Serves 5-6 dozen candies (40 servings)

Ingredients

11 ounce bag Kraft Caramel Bits (9g carbs package)

16 ounces white almond bark or candy melts

4 cups chocolate chips

3 cups walnuts or other nuts

1/2 cup extra white almond bark for drizzle

Directions

1. Prepare the almond bark to the size of chocolate chips if using, then put the walnuts in a 4 quart slow cooker while ensuring that you cover the bottom of cooking pot.

2. Then layer chocolate chips on the nuts, and follow with the almond bark.

3. Cover the crockpot and cook the ingredients on low settings for about 1 to 2 hours. To test for readiness, simply use a spoon to press the chocolate bark on top to check if about half of the chocolate has melted.

4. At this point, turn of the slow cooker and gently stir the mixture using a spatula or wooden spoon until the chocolate is smooth.

5. Then spoon the crockpot candy in spoonfuls into wax paper lined tray or paper lined mini muffin trays. You can use a medium cookie scoop to portion the candies too.

6. Now melt the remaining almond bark (for drizzle) based on package direction. Drizzle the melted almond bark over the candles with a spoon.

7. Allow the candy to cool down fully then store it in an airtight container.

Nutritional Information Per Serving: *Calories 200, Carbs 11g, protein 13.2g, Fat 16g*

Crème Brûlée

Prep Time 5 minutes

Cook Time 2 hours

Total Time 2 hours 5 minutes

Serves 12

Ingredients

1/4 of a vanilla bean

1/4 cup sugar, plus 2 teaspoons

1/2 cup heavy whipping cream

3 large egg yolks

Directions

1. Mix together whipping cream, egg yolks and a ¼ cup of sweetener if you want it. Whisk the ingredients until well combined.

2. Scrape the seeds from vanilla bean using a dull knife and then add about 1/8 teaspoon of vanilla bean seeds to the egg and cream mixture.

3. Whisk to blend and set aside. Get two 12 inch pieces of foil and roll them to resemble "a snake". Roll the snake shaped foil into a circle, while pinching the ends together.

4. Put the circular foil in the bottom of a crockpot and repeat the process with the second foil. Then put each of the ramekins on individual foil ring.

5. Add in boiling water to the crockpot, without splashing it on your custards. Ensure that the water reaches around one-third up the ramekins.

6. Set the crockpot to low setting and cook until the custard is cooked through, or for about 2 hours to 2 and a half hours. Poke the custard with a knife to test for doneness.

7. Now cover and keep it chilled for more than 6 hours. To serve, sprinkle with 2 teaspoons of your favorite sweetener and torch until brown.

Nutritional Information Per Serving: *Calories 103, Carbs 1g, Protein 2.3g, Fat 10g*

Chocolate Chip Brownie Cake

Prep Time: 15 minutes

Cook Time: 1 hour 30 minutes

Total Time: 1 hour 45 minutes

Serves 24

Ingredients

1/4 cup water

4 eggs

1/2 cup melted butter

1 packet chocolate chip cookie mix

1 box fudge brownies mix

Directions

1. Coat a crockpot with baking spray and set aside.

2. Then mix together 2 eggs, ¼ cup melted butter, the brownie mi along with water in a mixing bowl.

3. Stir the mixture well until blended then set aside.

4. Mix together ¼ cup of butter, chocolate chip cookie mix and eggs in a different mixing bowl. Stir to incorporate.

5. At this point, drop the brownie butter into the crockpot in spoonfuls until done. Cover and cook until it's no longer gooey in the center, or for about 1.5 to 2 hours.

6. Serve the brownie cake warm with whipped cream or ice cream.

Nutritional Information Per Serving: *Calories 152, Carbs 10g, Protein 11.6g, Fat 13.2g*

Cherry Dump Cake

Prep Time: 15 minutes

Cook Time: 2 hours

Total Time: 2 hours 15 minutes

Serves 24

Ingredients

42 ounce cherry pie filling

½ cup melted butter

1 box yellow cake mix

Directions

1. Mix the cake mix and melted butter in a bowl until well blended.

2. Grease the crockpot and then spread cherries from both cans in to the bottom of the cooking pot.

3. Crumble the mixture over the cherries and cover the ingredients. Cook on low for 4 hours or on high setting for approximately 2 hours.

Nutritional Information Per Serving: *Calories 100, Carbs 4g, Protein 6g, Fat 7.4g*

Caramel Apple Spice Cake

Prep Time: 15 minutes

Cook Time: 2 hours

Total Time: 2 hours 15 minutes

Serves 24

Ingredients

1/2 cup melted butter 1 stick

1 box Spice cake mix like Betty Crocker

2 tablespoons caramel sauce

1 teaspoon ground cinnamon

1/3 cup coconut palm sugar

4 large apples peeled and sliced

Vanilla ice cream or whipped cream for topping

Directions

1. Coat a crockpot with cooking spray. Then add in cinnamon, apples and the sweetener to the slow cooker and toss to coat the ingredients. Add in caramel and stir.

2. Sprinkle the Spice cake mix on the apples and distribute evenly a little of melted butter.

3. Cover the crockpot and cook until the fruit is bubbling and the top is somehow golden brown.

4. Serve the cake warm topped with vanilla ice cream or whipped cream topping.

Nutritional Information Per Serving: *Calories 61, Carbs 6g, Protein 6.4g, Fat 6.7g*

Caramel Cake

Prep Time: 15 minutes

Cook Time: 3 hours

Total Time 3 hours 15 minutes

Servings 8 -10

Ingredients

2 tablespoons butter

3/4 cup coconut palm sugar

1 1/2 cups boiling water

3 eggs

1/2 cup vegetable oil

1 cup Vanilla

1 approximately 15 ounce yellow cake mix

Directions

1. Coat a large crockpot with cooking spray or line it with a liner then coat with the spray.

2. Then in a large bowl, stir together eggs, oil, creamer and cake mix using a hand mixer or a whisk until smooth.

3. Place the mixture in the sprayed crockpot and set aside.

4. Meanwhile, in a small saucepan or heat-safe pan, bring some water to a boil then whisk in butter and the sweetener. Gradually drizzle the mixture over the cake batter.

5. Cover the slow cooker using a paper towel to help arrest any condensation that could otherwise wet the cake.

6. Cover the crockpot and cook at high setting approximately 2 hours. Start checking for doneness after 1 hour 30 minutes.

7. You can also insert a toothpick at a point where the cake mix doesn't resemble batter anymore. Some of the crumbs should also stick to the toothpick once cooked through.

8. Serve the caramel cake with ice cream and caramel sauce. Keep it in the fridge for not more than 3 days.

Nutritional Information Per Serving: *Calories 443, Carbs 5g, Protein 8.3g, Fat 19g*

Buttery Ranch Mushrooms

Prep Time: 5 minutes

Cook Time: 3 hours

Total Time: 3 hours 5 minutes

Serves 8

Ingredients

1 packet of dry ranch dressing mix

1/2 cup butter, melted

1 lb. fresh whole button mushrooms

1-2 tablespoons fresh parsley minced (optional, for garnish)

Directions

1. Thoroughly clean the mushrooms and then put them in a crockpot.

2. Whisk melted butter and dressing mix in a bowl, and then pour over the mushrooms the slow cooker. Stir well.

3. Cover the crockpot and cook on low setting for around 3 hour or so. Check if cooked through or cook for a few more minutes if you like.

4. Garnish the mushroom with fresh parsley as per you choice.

Nutritional Information Per Serving: *Calories 305, Carb 4g, Protein 7.7g, Fat 25g*

Conclusion

We have come to the end of the book. Thank you for reading and congratulations for reading until the end.

It's my sincere hope that this Ketogenic Crockpot recipe book has been of much help to you.

If you found the book valuable, can you recommend it to others? One way to do that is to post a review on Amazon.

Don't forget to leave a review for this book on Amazon!

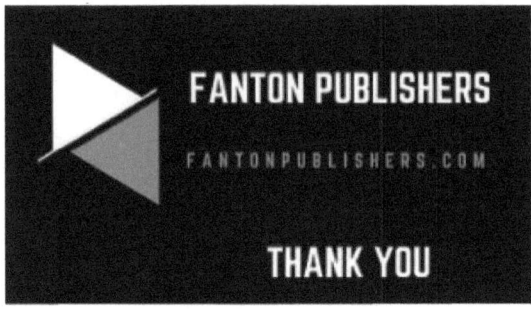

Do You Like My Book & Approach To Publishing?

If you like my writing and style and would love the ease of learning literally everything you can get your hands on from Fantonpublishers.com, I'd really need you to do me either of the following favors.

1: First, I'd Love It If You Leave a Review of This Book on Amazon.

2: Check Out My Other Keto Diet Books

KETOGENIC DIET: Keto Diet Made Easy: Beginners Guide on How to Burn Fat Fast With the Keto Diet (Including 100+ Recipes That You Can Prepare Within 20 Minutes)- New Edition

KETOGENIC DIET: Ketogenic Diet Recipes That You Can Prepare Using 7 Ingredients and Less in Less Than 30 Minutes

Ketogenic Diet: With A Sustainable Twist: Lose Weight Rapidly With Ketogenic Diet Recipes You Can Make Within 25 Minutes

Ketogenic Diet: Keto Diet Breakfast Recipes

Fat Bombs: Keto Fat Bombs: 50+ Savory and Sweet Ketogenic Diet Fat Bombs That You MUST Prepare Before Any Other!

Snacks: Keto Diet Snacks: 50+ Savory and Sweet Ketogenic Diet Snacks That You MUST Prepare Before Any Other!

Desserts: Keto Diet Desserts: 50+ Savory and Sweet Ketogenic Diet Desserts That You MUST Prepare Before Any Other!

Ketogenic Diet: Ketogenic Diet Lunch and Dinner Recipes

Ketogenic Diet: Keto Diet Cookbook For Vegetarians

Ketogenic Diet: Ketogenic Slow Cooker Cookbook: Keto Slow Cooker Recipes That You Can Prepare Using 7 Ingredients Or Less

Note: This list may not represent all my Keto diet books. You can check the full list by visiting my Author Central: amazon.com/author/fantonpublishers or my website http://www.fantonpublishers.com

Get updates when we publish any book on the Ketogenic diet: http://bit.ly/2fantonpubketo

Closely related to the keto diet is intermittent fasting. I also publish books on Intermittent Fasting.

One of the books is shown below:

Intermittent Fasting: A Complete Beginners Guide to Intermittent Fasting For Weight Loss, Increased Energy, and A Healthy Life

Get updates when we publish any book on intermittent fasting: http://bit.ly/2fantonbooksIF

To get a list of all my other books, please fantonwriters.com, my author central or let me send you the list by requesting them below: http://bit.ly/2fantonpubnewbooks

3: Let's Get In Touch

Antony

Website: http://www.fantonpublishers.com/

Email: Support@fantonpublishers.com

Twitter: https://twitter.com/FantonPublisher

Facebook Page: https://www.facebook.com/Fantonpublisher/

My Ketogenic Diet Books Page: https://www.facebook.com/pg/Fast-Keto-Meals-336338180266944

Private Facebook Group For Readers: https://www.facebook.com/groups/FantonPublishers/

Pinterest: https://www.pinterest.com/fantonpublisher/

4: Grab Some Freebies On Your Way Out; Giving Is Receiving, Right?

I gave you 2 freebies at the start of the book, one on general life transformation and one about the Ketogenic diet. Grab them here if you didn't grab them earlier.

Ketogenic Diet Freebie: http://bit.ly/2fantonpubketo

5 Pillar Life Transformation Checklist: http://bit.ly/2fantonfreebie

5: Suggest Topics That You'd Love Me To Cover To Increase Your Knowledge Bank. I am looking forward to seeing your suggestions and insights; you could even suggest improvements to this book. Simply send me a message on Support@fantonpublishers.com.

PSS: Let Me Also Help You Save Some Money!

If you are a heavy reader, have you considered subscribing to Kindle Unlimited? You can read this and millions of other books for just $9.99 a month)! You can check it out by searching for Kindle Unlimited on Amazon!

www.ingramcontent.com/pod-product-compliance
Lightning Source LLC
Chambersburg PA
CBHW030155100526
44592CB00009B/283